The Power of "Now" Unleashed!

How to set your Mind into Taking Action "Now" so you can achieve your Dreams

Melanie Hutchinson

Table of Contents

Introduction

Welcome and thank you for downloading this book; *"The Power of 'Now'"!*

This book contains proven steps and strategies on how to realize your dreams and accomplish them by taking action *today*.

Every person knows how to dream, but not all are willing to take the first and most important step towards their aspirations. Too many factors (*fear of failures, procrastination, disorganization*, and so on) can prevent even the most determined individual from taking a shot on their greatest ambitions.

In this book, you will learn fundamental lessons and strategies that will make you realize and adapt the *Power of 'Now'* for overcoming your doubts and pushing yourself towards success. These lessons include:

- *Realizing your core values and setting your direction for a meaningful life*

- *Finding the ultimate motivations for pushing yourself forward*

- *Getting more done by focusing on the present*

- *Managing your time for sustained productivity*

- *Overcoming doubts and worries*

- *And many more!*

Get Started NOW

The life you are living now – it is the only chance you will ever get. This is your one and only shot for the best life you can ever achieve. These statements may be simple, but they convey one of the most powerful messages ever. Do not pass up on this chance. Realize the *Power of 'Now'* and start living your life today!

Again, thank you for downloading this book and I hope you enjoy it!

Chapter 1:
Realizing your Dreams & Setting your Goals

"Having a vision and finding a direction is better than simply setting life goals."

Not a lot of people realize that identifying your dreams and goals is actually a crucial important "life skill". Dreams, ideals, goals, and purpose do not come out of nowhere. A person needs to learn how to look deep inside his own being to come up with these things.

Very few people have figured out exactly what they want for the future. This is because most of them are too busy looking for a "purpose" from all the wrong places. When in reality, they only need to identify what they really want. This is to find a direction; a direction that will lead to a brilliant future.

Remember that no one or nothing else has the power over your future. The future is not meant to be predicted – it is *created*. This is your own life, so you should create your own future.

The First Step

So, how exactly do you create your own future? Some will say that it starts with setting clear, specific goals; but there's more to it than you think. In the teachings of many life coaches, business gurus, authors, and other famous people, the importance of having a *life vision* is often overlooked. Let's face it; this is probably not your first time to think about your life goals *or* sought some form of guide to help you with them.

Here's a harsh fact; you can never really come up with a foolproof plan of achieving your long-term goals. There is also no reliable way to say that the things you want now will still be the things you want in the future. A mistake that a lot of people make is to waste time planning and figuring out everything before even taking the first step. But with a vision, you can focus more on getting started AND feeling fulfilled today.

Most of the time, you hear the advice; *"Be very specific with what you want in the future"*. This is actually a sound advice, but there is one problem. There is not enough emphasis on mustering enough courage to start the journey – which should begin *now*. Remember that you need to focus first on the journey before you can ever reach your destination. And this is what this book is all about – setting aside all doubts and stepping out the door.

Don't get this all wrong – you still need to identify your specific long-term goals. But before you set those goals, you need to identify first your vision. To prevent wasting any more time, you should start a *personal journal* to get to know yourself a little better.

Getting Started

Keeping a personal journal to create plans and track progress is nothing new in the professional world. If you do not have one, it is recommended that you acquire one as soon as possible. You can choose to keep a physical journal (*planner, notebook, etc.*) or use a computer application (*Evernote, Microsoft OneNote, etc.*). The answer depends on your personal preference. Just make sure you will have no trouble keeping your personal journal secure and private.

On the first page of your physical journal, write down a *self-introduction*. Use the template below and fill in the blanks to get started with this step:

My name is _____, age _____ and living in _____.

I currently work/study at _____ as a _____.

Feel free to include additional details regarding your relationships, education, and so on. If you've experienced writing a blog or work in a job that involves writing, then you'll know that everyone has their own "writing voice". If not, just write as if you're talking to the "future you" and it will come naturally.

Next comes the important part. In identifying your vision, you need to identify your *core values*. These values are your positive characteristics or beliefs that you can be proud of. These beliefs may benefit others or centered towards your personal growth. Here are some examples:

- *I like to learn more and perfect my abilities*

- *I want to see and experience the world*

- *I enjoy teaching young children*

- *I enjoy sharing my skills and talents*

- *I love to perform public service*

- *I like to help others solve their problems*

Remember that core values represent your deepest and sincerest beliefs. There is no special or strict rule when setting core values. Just bear in mind that they will be the main "driving force" that you should pursue. Also feel free to acknowledge as many core values as you want. Just make sure they are sincere. These values, in turn, will fuel you with motivation for your long-term goals.

Believe it or not, identifying your core values will also make you feel better about your life later on. Businesses and organizations even uphold their own "visions" or "value statements" to help members/employees work towards a single direction.

Why is this important to you? Because core values essentially help you create better decisions that lead to results you will most likely be thankful for. Core values do more than your individual skills and talents in terms of fulfillment. For example, if you particularly enjoy teaching others, then you should feel rewarded simply by getting the opportunity to share your knowledge. Regardless if a goal succeeds or not, you will still feel "enriched". And this is probably the greatest lesson you will ever learn in goal setting.

Setting Long-term Goals

Now that you've identified your core values, you can now set long-term goals that suit you perfectly. Don't forget to consider your skills, talents, and passions when setting long-term goals. Remember that abilities – innate or learned – are some of the greatest assets that can give you great success.

Just like in the world of business, you need to follow your own passions and carve your own path. And by incorporating your core values, you are more likely to stick to your direction in the long run. This is the ultimate combination for accomplishing anything you can dream of.

Remember that you only need to fulfill at least one of your core values *in the process* if you wish to incorporate them into a goal. For example, if your long-term goal is to become a world-renowned business coach and entrepreneur, then a matching core value could be to *share the secrets of success with others.*

Without further ado, it's time to set your long-term goals. On your personal journal, create a list of the **5-10**greatest long-term goals you can think of. These will be the things you're looking to accomplish within the next 3-10 years. With such a long timeframe, there is no reason for you to set lesser goals and undermine your own abilities. Always *think big* without being unrealistic. You may also set materialistic goals as long as they align to your core values.

To keep things simple, set long-term goals using only *1-2 sentences* per goal. No need to write entire paragraphs or include in-depth plans. Just make sure to determine how your core values are incorporated with each of your goals.

The obstacle you should worry about now is finding the motivation to actually start your life journey. In short, you only need to actually have a *visualization* of the finish line.

Creating a Motivation Collage

To wrap up everything you've learned in this chapter, you can create a "motivation collage" to help maintain a clear picture of your long-term goals. It is also regarded as a simple, yet effective productivity tool for a quick boost of motivation.

Basically, a motivation collage is a collection of images or other visual articles that represent your long-term goals. It could be a picture of your dream car, your dream house, a view from your dream vacation, and so on.

Just like with your core values, there should be no strict rule in creating your own collage. You can make it as big as a poster or as small as a card in your wallet. The easiest way to create a motivation collage is to perform an *image search* on the internet and paste/attach them to a single document.

Chapter 2:
Start Focusing on the 'Now'

"If you want to take action today, you need to live in the present."

After identifying your core values and setting your long-term goals, you are one step closer to figuring out how to get there. But first, you need to learn how to live in the present not just physically, but mentally and emotionally as well. For this chapter, it is important for you to remain focused and collected as you *reconnect with the present*. This can be done using a few strategies that allow you to think objectively and build your confidence.

Reconnecting with the Present

Keep in mind that the title of this book is "The Power of *Now*" – not "The Power of Yesterday" or "The Power of Tomorrow".

The only part of your life you should be worried about is neither the past nor the future– it is the present. The past is for learning, the future is for aspiring, and the present is for *acting*. Keep in mind that the present is your only opportunity to take action. Unfortunately, some people waste this opportunity by thinking about the past and worrying about the future.

Why is this so important in accomplishing your goals? Here are some of the most important reasons:

- **Removing Worry** – Remember that pondering in the future or past introduces a sense of being powerless. This leads to needless worry and unnecessary stress, which can be easily be avoided by reconnecting with the present.

- **Better Focus** —Reconnecting with the present is the only way for you to gain clarity and focus. Remember that these two things are crucial for productivity and progress.

- **Getting Things Done** —Snapping back to the present is of utmost importance especially if you are the type of person who likes to delay responsibilities and set them aside for *tomorrow*.

- **Better Decisions** – Thoughts from the past and worries from the future can sometimes cloud your judgment. If you want to make better decisions, you need to liberate yourself from these psychological distractions.

- **Better Experience and Learning** – Do not miss the opportunity to learn valuable lessons by present experiences. In the next chapter, you will learn more about the importance of experience in accomplishing goals and achieving your dreams.

The premise of reconnecting with the present is easier said than done. Nevertheless, it is an essential step to take before you can focus on *how* you will accomplish your goals. Now that you've learned the benefits of focusing on the present, you should be able to notice that it is more on eliminating distractions and cultivating your focus on what you need to do *today*.

Without noticing, a lot of people have imprinted worry as a normal part of their busy lifestyle. They worry about the bills, anticipate the stress of future work, and think about undesirable events that are yet to happen or won't even happen at all. Furthermore, they let mistakes in the past distract them from what really matters; which is the present.

With this being said, here are some simple strategies that can help you snap back to the present:

Create a daily 'To-Do' List

Staying organized with your tasks for the current day is a great practice to focus on the present. Upon receiving or identifying the tasks for today (from *work, school,* or *business*), make it a habit to write them down sequentially. Aside from being ahead of your daily objectives, having a to-do list also provides a sense of accomplishment upon the completion of one task.

There are many useful tools and software applications you can use to create a to-do list. One of the simplest ways is to use *Sticky Notes,* which is a desktop application that lets you write short notes quickly. Other good alternatives are post-it notes, a planner notebook, or straight into your personal journal. In the next chapter, you will find a comprehensive guide on how to prioritize daily objectives more effectively.

Write on your Personal Journal daily

In the previous chapter, you learned the importance of keeping a personal journal for being more in touch with your core values. Your personal journal is one of the very few places wherein you can communicate with yourself; helping you to assess and reflect on your daily decisions along the way. But most importantly, your personal journal is one of the best tools you have for tracking important events and progress in your daily life.

A simple practice to help you focus more on the present is to record your relevant experiences and thoughts at least once a day. This is best done during the night right before going to sleep. Also remember that you can write in any tone or style you wish on your personal journal.

If you're keeping a personal planner, do not forget to include the current date as you write. Lastly, use a highlighter pen to emphasize relevant things and try to review those things the day after.

Use a Calendar and mark future events

Despite being widely used in workplaces and most homes, some people can still forget the current date. With the modern lifestyle, you sometimes feel like it's sufficient just to know what day it is in the week. This mindset will eventually make you anticipate and long for Fridays while dreading the arrival of Mondays. Sounds familiar?

Another simple habit you can do to keep yourself in the present is to use a calendar. This is to simply look at the calendar every morning; that's it. Make use of all types of calendars you can find. It could be the calendar on your planner, on your smartphone, or the one hanging on your wall. All you need to do is to highlight the current date (or flip the page to the current date – depending on the type of calendar you're using) and mark future events within the month. You should also set reminders on important dates using calendars on your smartphone or computer.

Look for 1 Accomplishment Today

Remember that the ultimate purpose of reconnecting with the present moment is to find an opportunity to do something worthwhile. Every new day is literally filled with hundreds or even *thousands* of opportunities to make it relevant. In fact, just 1 accomplishment is enough to make your day count. All you need to do is to recognize and grab any of these opportunities. Here are some examples:

- *Perform or accomplish an incomplete work from the previous day*

- *Learn a new piece of music*

- *Finish reading a new self-help eBook*

- *Try a new recipe*

- *Repair something that has been broken for some time*

- *Work out or engage in a physical activity*

- *Get the number of the girl/boy you like*

- *Make peace with someone whom you've had a quarrel with*

- *Make a new friend or approach someone new from within your organization/community*

Again, there are virtually infinite ways to get something done today. Even if none of the examples above is available to you right now, you can aim to *improve* a previous accomplishment. Set new records and keep on breaking old ones. Contrary to popular belief, you don't really need to be always working towards your long-term dreams – not if you realize that every day fulfills a goal no matter how simple it may be.

Chapter 3:
Planning your Action

"If you know how to plan for the short-term, you're halfway of getting there."

With everything you've learned so far, you should now be able to realize the importance of having a direction and living in the present. These are two of the most important lessons that will make you realize how crucial every moment is to accomplishing your long-term goals. Next, you need to learn how to effectively set your short-term goals and manage your time. Take a deep breath because you're about to get your hands full in this chapter.

Applying S.M.A.R.T

One of the best popular methods of setting goals and objectives is to apply the *S.M.A.R.T criteria*. S.M.A.R.T stands for *Specific, Measurable, Assignable, Realistic,* and *Time-bound* in the world of business. It was originally formulated to help in employee-performance and project management in business leadership. But with a few changes in words (*A* for *Attainable* and *R* for *Resource-oriented*), it can also be helpful for personal development.

Here is an explanation for each element in the S.M.A.R.T criteria for personal development:

1. **Specific** – In setting objectives and short-term goals, you need to specify *what exactly* needs to be done and *who* will be the people involved. In contrast to long-term goals, you need as much details as possible and

prepare for every possible outcome. Be as in-depth as possible. Being specific greatly helps in managing risks and getting better results.

2. **Measurable** – To set objectives and goals more effectively, you need to be able to measure your progress for making changes and some adjustments. For example, say you need to raise $5,000 in 5 months for a business startup. Given these parameters, you need to raise at least $1,000 per month to meet your objective. But if you only managed to raise $800 in the first month, this means something in your fundraising strategy is not working and must be modified.

3. **Assignable (for Business)** –Assigning tasks to the most able person is one of the basic rules of project management. To effectively set goals for your organization, you need to specify and assign a set of tasks that will collectively complete an objective. Make sure that each member is contributing their fullest by considering both their strengths and weaknesses.

4. **Attainable (for Personal Development) or Realistic (for Business)**–For personal development, you need to set goals that you can realistically accomplish with your current capabilities. For this, you can come up with ideas that adapt to your previous accomplishments. Of course, you should also consider external factors (certain laws or regulations, current technology, etc.) that can limit the things you can actually accomplish.

5. **Resource-oriented (for Personal Development)** – Effectively managing and allocating resources is a given for business. But this is also important for

personal growth and development. Remember that for your personal goals, you are exclusively responsible for your own resources. Most personal goals require not only money, but time and energy as well to see progress. With this being said, be sure to manage your investments more wisely and carefully.

6. **Time-bound** – Lastly, each objective should come with specific *deadlines*. Applying this simple practice will give each task a degree of urgency that will almost guarantee completion. Additionally, setting deadlines is a crucial aspect of time management.

Managing your Time

Effective time management methods include creating a timetable, setting "time boxes" for completing tasks, and setting deadlines. Before anything, you need to at least have a weekly timetable to help you manage and organize your time. Timetables can be created on materials or software that can easily be edited. For example, a whiteboard or a spreadsheet document on your computer allows you to easily modify your timetable. With this being said, printing your timetable or writing it on a page in your personal journal may not be the best idea.

Creating a timetable should be relatively simple. Just create a table with column headings that refer to the days of the week (Monday, Tuesday, Wednesday ...). Next, create an iteration of your waking hours during the day on the leftmost column. Here is a simple example of a timetable:

	Mon	Tues	Wed	Thurs	Fri	*Sat*	*Sun*
7:00-8:00							
8:00-9:00							
9:00-10:00							
10:00-11:00							

Time Boxing

Time boxing is regarded by many professionals as the most effective time management tool for productivity. It is used for project management, agile software development, and risk management. It can also be used personally to set deadlines for individual objectives in a much quicker rate. Furthermore, organizing time boxes can help anyone improve focus and overcome procrastination.

You can integrate the time boxing technique with your weekly timetable. All you need to do is to specify what you need to accomplish by a set time. The most manageable time box length is *30 minutes,* which is enough to accomplish most small tasks without being too physically and mentally exhausting. Time boxing can also be effectively used with your daily to-do list (refer to previous chapter).

Here are additional tips for successful time boxing:

- **Include 30-minute breaks after 3 time boxes (90 minutes of work)** – Studies suggest that a person can only focus on productivity for 90 minutes before feeling tired. After 90 minutes of focused work, the brain sends "stress signals" such as hunger, drowsiness, and inattentiveness to tell you that it needs to take a break. To restore lost performance, full rest for 25-30 minutes should suffice.

- **Don't make it difficult** – One of the main problems of time boxing is setting unrealistic or extremely difficult deadlines. Be aware that time boxing can be a double-edged sword. If accomplishing the requirements in a time box is very rewarding, missing a deadline is very stressful. With this being said, it is important to learn how to effectively break down difficult tasks into smaller and more manageable "chunks". If you so require, you can opt for 1-hour time boxes to give yourself more room to breathe.

- **Time box for fun** – There is no realistic way for a person to load up on productivity without spending some time for recreation. It simply isn't possible to sustain that kind of lifestyle. With this being said, you may include a maximum of 3 hours in a day for activities that you enjoy.

- **Work on the hardest task first** –A common mistake that busy people make is to focus on the easy, less-relevant tasks first before starting with the more important ones. This is because the most relevant objectives are usually the hardest. Remember that doing this will not lessen the stress you will feel at the end of the day. In fact, you are more likely to experience more stress if you use up your energy on less important tasks first. This is why you should aim to complete the most important tasks first while your mind and body are still rested.

Make sure you already have your completed timetable. You may also start planning for the tasks you have for the rest of the week. This is optional. What's really important is for you to get started in the earliest time possible. If you simply cannot start today, you can start tomorrow but no later than that.

Chapter 4:
Eliminating Fear and Overcoming Worry

"Having a learner's mindset is the key for guaranteeing progress regardless if you succeed or not."

As stated in the first chapter, there is no point in coming with in-depth plans for long-term goals if you are yet to take your first step. It's not the lack of plans or confidence that prevents anyone from starting; it is the tendency to *overthink*.

The problem of having too many questions

It is normal for a person to have a ton of questions after setting an amazing goal or realizing an incredible dream. Although pondering in these questions encourages you to think deep, it is a probability that thinking a little *too deep* will lead to uncertainty and fear. Will you ever achieve your ultimate goals? Will you ever be a "somebody"? What if you can never accomplish any of your plans? What if you *fail*?

As fear and doubt develop deep inside you, you grow more and more hesitant to even take your first step. So instead of focusing on finding *all* the answers, you should focus on *experiencing the questions*.

Granted, it is quite easy to obtain knowledge and vital information through research and self-study nowadays, especially with the ever-expanding knowledge base that is the internet. You can even pay for the information you need through subscriptions, online courses, and professional coaching. This will, to an extent, diminish the risk of experiencing failure and may even give you a small boost of confidence.

But even so, no one else can really provide you with a 100% complete, step-by-step plan on how to get to exactly where you want to be in life. The knowledge and information you obtain from other sources will always "feel" insufficient as long as you haven't experienced them yet.

With all these being said, remember that the best way to learn is to *experience*. Failures, successes, accomplishments – all these are essentially forms of *discovery*. And by adapting this mindset, a significant part of the fear and uncertainty you're feeling should be gone by now.

Perfection is overrated

In the words of psychologist and bestselling author *Dr. Harriet B. Braiker; "Striving for excellence motivates you; striving for perfection is demoralizing."*

In other words, perfection in everything can be pursued, but it can never really be accomplished. When it comes to setting goals and objectives, no one can really come up with perfect plans. You can only start with imperfect plans with a direction that is *perfect* to you.

Remember that achieving perfection should not be your priority as you start. In fact, it shouldn't be your priority ever. If you achieve a state that you deem "perfect", you are effectively eliminating the possibility of learning something new. Keep in mind that there will always be room for improvement no matter how far you think you've come.

Simply adapting this mindset can make you less fearful of failures and more willing to take risks. Learning is, after all, one of the most valuable experiences anyone could have in life. If the world is perfect, it would be extremely boring. Strive to discover and learn from its imperfections instead.

The only thing you need to be ready is to *think* that you're ready. With this in mind, there should be absolutely no reason left to wait. Go out there, take chances, fail, succeed, learn, and make progress. If you're ready, move on to the next chapter.

Chapter 5:
Being Accountable

"You decide how you will be remembered by others."

Simply put, being accountable is the best way for you to motivate yourself if all else fails. But first, what does it really mean to be accountable?

Some would say that you should be accountable for the consequences of your actions. In business, a leader is always accountable for the entire team's failures. At first, being accountable seems like another source of motivation by pressuring yourself to do well. But being accountable should not be limited to the outcome. To be accountable, you need to assume the sole responsibility for all of your *choices*.

Why be accountable?

There is only one thing you need to do in order to be accountable. Go ahead and *tell someone* all that you've learned throughout this entire book. Every person in this planet has that "someone" they can rely on in terms of sharing these things. It could be your spouse, your sibling, your best friend, or your mentor.

You might think that it is a good strategy to keep your goals and objectives to yourself. After all, keeping these things private will make you less afraid to make mistakes. But sometimes, you need to let other people "in" to receive one of the most important assets anyone can get – *support*.

The more respectable your core values are, the more support you can get from people. This is another reason why it is important for you to identify your core values. And in addition to encouragement, you can also get feedback and vital input from the people who truly matter.

Finally, be sure to learn how to listen to criticism for they are more opportunities for learning. You can even ask for their help to get something accomplished faster. But most importantly, making someone else proud of your achievements is one of the most rewarding experiences in the world.

How to be accountable?

Other than the simple method described above, here are some more simple ideas on how to be accountable:

- Share accomplishments and failures with friends

- Join a discussion group about an interest that is related to your goals

- Offer your help or guidance to someone with the same interests as you

- Ask someone: *"What do you think?"*

- Be honest whenever you can

- Find people who can help you obtain a skill or quality that you lack

- Always admit your mistakes and exert some effort to make up for them

- Respect others

- *Respect yourself*

Chapter 6:
A Leap of Faith

"To live, to TRULY live, we must be willing to RISK. To be nothing in order to find everything. To leap before we look."

Often, people are presented with the opportunity to fulfill their dreams. Although this may seem ideal, and even like something that you want badly, it is often at these times that people freeze up and become indecisive. Rushing through their minds is information on all the risks involved, as well as fears and worry that things will not go according to plan. Although uncomfortable and unhappy in their current situation, they are comfortable enough to not want to change it too much. They often will back down from their dream as it seems impossible that it would be so easy to attain, and they are then left wondering 'what it', leading to the experience of misery for a large portion of their lives. At this point, they will look back with resignation, realizing that a lot of time was spent on activities that brought no joy.

There are so many reasons why a person would want to experience more of the same, rather than taking a leap of faith and actually trying to realize their dreams by living in the now. Take for example, you want to change careers so that you can do something you love, rather than stay in a job simply because you earn enough to pay the bills. You may refuse to move from your current position because it may affect your stability and comfort ability, in a few years' time you may qualify for a reward from your workplace for loyal service, your remuneration is barely meeting your needs and you cannot afford risk, you are receiving a whole range of additional benefits which you might not have access to if you make a change and so many other credible reasons. Your internal dialogue is doing a constant risk assessment to determine whether it is "safe" for you to follow your dreams. More often than not, your mind will highlight all the negative aspects of any plan, making you less likely to follow through on taking a leap of faith. So if you want to achieve your dreams, you need to shut off that voice in your head that will give you a myriad of reasons as to why you cannot, and just forget risk and take a leap of faith.

Understand Faith and How to take the Leap

Faith is simply defined as believing in the positivity that can come from the unseen. This believing is blind, and should be wholeheartedly expressed to be used within the understanding of faith. Taking a leap of faith is therefore the act of leaping into the unseen and the unknown, with the belief that things will work out so that you can reach your desired end result. When you go blindly into the unknown, you do not have the opportunity to prepare to address any arising scenarios. A leap of faith may entail making a risky decision, which would involve a certain amount of sacrifice on your part, even if you have evaluated all the alternatives and it appears that they are not going to work in your favor. It is all about following your gut feeling to attain a particular result. It entails letting go of fear and doubt, so that you can experience the unknown.

There is a saying that states "Fool me once, shame on me. Fool me twice, shame on me." If you want to fulfill your dreams now, but feel as though you are stuck in a rut, you will need to evaluate your behaviors now. Look at your daily routine and identify what practices you repeat for than once in a day. Then review those practices to identify which ones give you joy, which ones give you income and so on. If one is consistently repeating the same action and expecting a different result is not conducive in their actions and beliefs.

You should consider taking a leap of faith now. In that, you can decide whether you are going to take a large leap which is highly significant, or whether you were going to take a smaller leap that is more practical and functional. It can be something small or it could be large and highly significant. If you are working in a shop as a supervisor, and you dream of being permanently financially stable, you could try a small leap of faith like asking your superior for higher wages, or you would try something more extreme like leaving your current job, putting together your savings and starting that culinary venture that you have always dreamed of.

As the leap of faith entails some sacrifice, it also requires a generous dose of courage. When the payoff in any situation appears to be more than the cost of maintaining the status quo, then a leap of faith is easier to carry out.

A leap of faith is perhaps the most likely immediate action you can take to fulfill your dreams. Leaping entails taking a big jump, and making a bold decision now will involve you having to take that first step. Once you have passed this test, then you need to consciously make an effort to visualize your leap of faith, and then take it. You can only ever make a successful leap of faith if you fully believe in yourself, and in your abilities to address any situation that is presented to you face on.

Chapter 7:
Get Inspiration from Others

"The good life is one inspired by love and guided by knowledge".

The world is full of billions of people, and each person is completely unique. Different people have different opinions, behaviors and methods of being. When looking to get inspiration from somewhere, you can try your luck attracting the attention of someone in a full room. If they are looking to establish a friendship, you can take the opportunity to listen to what they have to say just in case it inspires you in some way.

Should you have an opportunity to speak to someone about fulfilling dreams and living their ideal life, you are likely to also hear a description of someone that they admire. This person that they admire may be someone who has already managed to attain the dreams that they are looking towards. It could also be someone who has fulfilled some dream and become successful. They are living that ideal lifestyle, whether it is that they have acquired a certain amount of material belongings, or they have received fame and recognition for their hard work, or even that they have become experts in what they do so they are the 'go to' people for a job. Whatever the reason, the person that is admired is often given a name to reflect the given admiration and put them into context. These people may be referred to as mentors, inspirers, leaders, and a whole range of other titles.

The Power of the Mentor in your Life

If you want to set your mind into taking action now so that you can achieve your dreams as you have seen with a mentor, then you need to make sure that you choose the right person to emulate, someone who inspires you. You can then mold yourself towards their behavior and character. The reason that this step is critical is because there are a range of people who appear to be more than what they really are.

The most inspiring people are those who have fulfilled their dreams through some effort on their part. Their efforts could include solid hard work; a brilliant idea that transformed their situation in life, a leap of faith that they took that paid off in the long run, or evens a stroke of good fortune which has been masterfully handled so that they can reap from available benefits. Rags to riches stories in particular are the most impressionable and inspirational.

Once you have identified your mentor, you need to study them extremely deeply. Get to know about the different aspects of the personalities, and how these contributed to their current success. Review their lifestyle, and even look at how they treat the people around them. Identify the steps that were taken to attain success, and analyses any underlying processes that may have been used for reference purposes. You may find that they have identified rock solid ways or developed motivating behaviors that you can imitate to help you powerfully take action now to fulfill your dreams. This type of analysis will allow you to have a holistic view of your mentors, so that you can choose to imitate the best parts of their personas.

By looking at the actions that your mentor took, you can set your mind to positive and inspirational thoughts. Many times we are our own greatest enemy, simply because we speak negativity into our situation or circumstance. Observing your mentor should give you the tools to change your mind set from negativity, where you judge your circumstances or those around you harshly, to positively viewing the good things in your situation and identifying how others can help so that good things can happen in your life. When you judge or criticize yourself or others, you drain your energy both mentally and physically, making it impossible for you to act in the now.

As well as finding your mentor from a pool of people that you know and admire, you might try to do so by talking with a complete stranger. The Power of now supports spontaneity and opening your mind to new experiences can go quite a way when you are trying to fulfill your dreams. In addition, meeting with a stranger and discussing things with strangers may present the opportunity to bounce of ideas from someone who may oppose your natural train of thought. This kind of interaction can help you assess how your mind works, and whether you are being present enough to people.

Break away from Negativity

Having negative thoughts and acting on them is something that is often done at the subconscious level. Your judgment and criticism of yourself and of others may be so in built in your mind that you are not even aware of the times that you are being negative. So when you are viewing someone more fortunate that you are, rather than begrudging them their belongings or feeling high levels of envy, you can use the power of now to speak positivity into the situation. You could use these successful inspiring people as your personal inspiration, and work on making some affirmative statements to yourself such as "Just like my mentor, I can figure out how they have become so successful, and I can create a template that works for me."

One person who has been able to live in the power of now is Bill Gates. As he disburses money from sales, as well as to his charity that supports projects all over the world. While doing these activities, he can only focus on the now, what is being done and when he will be affected. Emulating his thought process is more than likely what is needed when trying to elevate to the next level.

Once you make the decision to allow yourself to draw inspiration from others, that you gain your own significant amount of power while prompting you into taking immediate action to fulfill your dreams. You also learn methods that you can use to expand your creativity, so that should a need arise; it can be addressed from your location easily.

Chapter 8:
Failure is Success

"Being able to recognize a failure just means that you'll be able to re-cast it into something more likely to succeed."

Many people are working towards attaining success. It is important to understand that success is as a result of overcoming many barriers as well as picking yourself up after extended periods of failure. Although success if something that people seem to work towards achieving in the future, it still remains very relevant to gradually ensuring that you can utilize the power of now.

Failure is one of those words that always brings about a dampening of moods, a little sadness and perhaps even some despondence. It is understood as something that happens that you should be ashamed of. It reflects on your effort for a particular task, and failure may be unfairly translated as laziness. When one hears about failure, they immediately lose motivation and concentration, and if possible, they will do everything that they possibly can to avoid this feeling entirely.

Once you choose to start or to follow the path to accomplishing your dreams, you are likely to make many mistakes. If you stumble and fall, you must try, and try, and try again. You see, failure offers you the very best opportunity to set your mind to taking action. This happens when you can train your brain to recognize failure as a simple stepping stone or learning curve on your journey.

Using Failure for Positive Purposes

For failure to be effective, you must also react to it in the right way. You should avoid going into denial, so much so that he would refuse to do so. In addition, make sure that you do not start chasing all your losses or crying over spilled milk. Both of these situations can easily be dealt with. Failure needs someone who is flexible, and able to adjust their plans if necessary. When you are faced with an equation for example that you just cannot seem to work out, getting upset and physically abusive with the family pet will not change the fact that you failed at a task.

Failure allows you to become conscious of the many ways that you may be holding yourself back. You may have attempted to carry out a tasked and failed publicly, leading to a feeling of shame. Or it could be that you have submitted a proposal several times and it always comes back without you receiving a good pass. Taking action now will help take your mind off your losses, where your mind can fester, think all sorts of things, and stop working as effectively as it did before. When things of this nature happen, it also gives the families the opportunity to try new things.

With an increased sense of awareness, you can analyses a range of situations, as well as make improvements to your already exiting issues. You should never view failure as something negative because failure is success. Failure reveals that you are taking steps towards achieving your goals, because if you never tried, then you would be left with nothing to show for it at all. However, you might find yourself getting frustrated if the more you try; the less likely it appears that you will be able to succeed. If this frustration occurs, do not panic and most importantly, do not give up. You have the power and the insight to gain complete control of your mind, and it is at these instances that you should share wisdom and healthy decision making. As you experience failure, you should learn the lessons you need to learn along the way, but never use these lessons as an excuse to keep you away from achieving your dreams starting now.

Your attitude to failure should be that you are clear about the end result, but undecided about the method. Sometimes when you fail, it is not because of trying or getting the steps wrong, it is about how we are trying to learn the steps and get the situation right. You should view failure as a "bump in the road".

Failure also helps with your clarity about what you really need to be doing in order to be successful. You might have to move to a different town, or tap in to a separate plan, or change the materials that you are using for executing a project. In addition to offering clarity, one need a healthy dose of patience as it may take some time to adequately overcome failure.

When you are setting your mind towards achieving success and fulfilling your dreams, you should never feel sorry for yourself if things should go wrong, or veer of the plan. Remember that failure is not a reflection of who you are as a person; rather failure reveals to you what you are doing wrong to achieve your dreams. Failure is more about the actions that you have taken, rather than your overall character.

Before you declare that you have finally accomplished the elusive success, make sure that you get feedback from as many people as possible. When you view failure as success, it helps you maintain your confidence as you need to believe that your failures are surmountable. You must believe in yourself and keep our head up while moving forward.

Chapter 9:
Get Rid of the Hurdles in your Way

"A hero is an ordinary individual who finds the strength to persevere and endure in spite of overwhelming obstacles".

When you picture a hurdle, you are likely to imagine something that you find at a sporting arena. These are those barriers that are put in the path of an athlete and in order to get past them, the athlete has to take a high jump over them. They are meant to avoid hitting these hurdles and toppling them over during a race. Though these hurdles seem to capture the essence of what a hurdle could be, hurdles include much more than that. So far, there are several hurdles that have been discussed in this book. These include the hurdles of fear and worry. There are a myriad of other hurdles that you are likely to encounter as you work towards living in the present and achieving your dreams. These hurdles are likely to slow you down, stress you out with numerous demands and while playing on your own limited knowledge, and discourage you at every turn; that is until you find a way to overcome them.

To identify these hurdles, you need to look at the present situation and figure out a way that you can try to make your dreams come to life. So ask yourself the following questions: -

a) What is keeping you from fulfilling your dreams right now, from this moment on?

b) Are you surrounding yourself with people who cannot see or translate your vision, and therefore they put your down and discourage you?

c) Have you spent so much time at an unfulfilling job?

d) Are you doing anything in excess in your life, such as overeating, drinking too much alcohol, or using narcotics?

e) Do you find yourself stuck, and unable to pinpoint what is keeping you this way?

Once you have answered these questions, you will be able to make you out exactly what your hurdles are, and a deeper understanding of the hurdles should reveal ways in which you can overcome them. The answers could be varied, but generally speaking, if you can acknowledge that any of these situations are having an effect on your life, then you are facing a hurdle.

The hurdles that are most prevalent, and that can stop you from fulfilling your dreams and taking action in the now include: -

- **Financial Hurdles** – This involves taking an honest look at your finances and making a decision to spend in a certain way. The biggest hurdle here that stops people from living in the now is the credit card. So you would need to destroy your credit cards and use cash. A credit card has you living in the past or in the future especially in regards to the payments. In the past in that you have to pay for things where you spend money that you do not already have, and in the future where you are anticipating how much more you can spend of the money that you do not already have. Not having a credit card solves the problem of irrational spending and is good to remove the hurdle that bad financing can have on your overall self.

- **Meeting Urgency** – There are many times when you are at your workplace and the boss comes in requesting for some urgent work to be done. Usually you will hear the words drop everything and you then work based on urgency rather than proper planning. This type of hurdle has you looking into the past, as there will always be work that had to be left behind so that the urgent tasks could be completed. It also interrupts your organization, and can throw a spanner in the works when you are trying to accomplish a goal. You should make a stand in regards to your work, and find a balance between working under pressure of urgency and consistently following through on your already developed plan.

- **Exercise Hurdles** – Keeping fit is part and parcel of stimulating your mind. It is also the type of activity that cannot be stowed away until later. When working, the one thing that many shirk on is exercises. It might seem odd that exercise can help you achieve your dreams now, but a mind that is alert and able to take in information, is much better than one that is sluggish, especially if you need to make important decisions that could alter your life or a situation. Exercise helps to prepare your body for the decisions that your mind will make to take action now.

When you start to get rid of these hurdles, you may find that you hurt someone emotionally or that you inconvenience them. This may make you feel guilty, deterring you from working on these hurdles. If you are unable to get rid of these hurdles, it means that you have made the decision to not focus on the power of now and all the benefits that it offers. You have put yourself last, instead of valuing yourself enough to make your dreams come true.

Overcoming hurdles also involves refocusing your mind to the now. You need to consistently and with determination focus your mind on the present, so that some of your hurdles will slowly chance completely. Tackling your hurdles one at a time is the best way to live in the now.

What you can do is take some time to list all of your hurdles that you feel may be affecting your ability to move forward or live in the present. Also, include any hurdles that may be dragging you into the past. Then go through this list, eliminating them from your life systematically until you have no hurdles left.

Chapter 10:
Appreciate your abilities

"Appreciate your abilities and trust your instincts. Just because you haven't done something doesn't mean you can't."

There is one mindset that we all experience when we are trying to accomplish something and that is doubt – a little seed of doubt goes a long way in stopping you from the power of now and using your abilities to accomplish all your dreams. When you are looking to set your mind towards achieving a dream, you can view your dream in the same way as that little seed. When you have a seed, you can grow it into the largest of trees and bushes. The small seeds will need to be nurtured and taken care of so that it can grow and bloom into something beautiful.

However, if you treat your dreams like you would a tree, and you have reached the point where the flowers are in bloom or the fruit is likely to be in season, you would not let anything come in the way of getting the last out of that tree. It is like running in a race and then seeing the finish line. If it was a marathon, you are sure to find the renewed strength that you will need to barrel through. When you have doubt, you need to avoid cultivating the seed, because if you do so, you will not appreciate the results which could bring you own. Doubt makes you consistently question your abilities to get something done in the right way, and what usually happens when you have doubt is that you do not do what needs to be done; you just manage enough to get by and hope that it will be acceptable.

Take Advantage of your Gifts, Talents or Ability

Every person has a free gift, talent or ability that is ingrained within them. When you want the power of now to be of an advantage to you, you need to mentally isolate your gift. This means that within your own mind, you should be able to identify your gift for what it is, and know how you can use it so that it is useful for you and can benefit others. You should apply your gift and build your confidence, knowing that you can do something worthwhile. Using gifts for the benefit of other people is an excellent way for you to live in the present. As each person has a different gift, you should not take your own gift for granted after you have made a comparison with the gifts of other people. Rather, you need to appreciate it, and figure out ways that you can bring the best out of your gift at all times. There is no lesser or better gift, just different ways that gifts can be used.

As you deal with a myriad of emotions and scenarios, it may be easy for you to believe that you may not have what it takes to complete every aspect of a project. That is fair thinking because it is unlikely that a carpenter has full marketing experience for example. When doing a project, certain skills may be required like communication skills, social skills and technical skills. If you have an ability to learn, you can get some basic training and start working. Embracing your abilities means that you really need to sit down and think about them. In addition, you should be able to actively use your mind so that you can build on them. This way, you become better and better at a range of things, allowing you to fit into more projects and situations. Appreciating your abilities should also include the benefits that you will enjoy by expanding on them.

You need to believe in your ability to work in the power of now. Through this book, a range of strategies had been discussed that all center on you believing within your mind that you can take action starting now – not tomorrow, not after due consideration, not after consultation with experts, but right now. These strategies all tie together with appreciation. Appreciation is the key to living in the now, as it is something that does not look too far into the past or into the future. Appreciation focuses on looking at what is happening in the now, and making an immediate decision on how it is making your life easier. It can help you easily see the different things that are coming together and happening in your life so that you can achieve your dreams. When you appreciate something, you are more likely to live in the moment as you try bringing it to fruition.

Another simple way of appreciating your abilities is to take some time to really look at your qualifications. What are you good at or what have you been trained in that can help you use the power of now? List all these qualities or qualifications down, and use this list to channel behavior that is conducive to making your dreams come true.

In addition, you should be clear about what you love and what you do not love. This type of clarity ensures that you do not waste your precious time putting stock into actions or activities that do not give you joy. When you do something you do not like, you are unlikely to approach it with the same passion as something you do like, and this in itself will have an effect on the final result that you are hoping to achieve.

When you appreciate your abilities, you also become a good role model for others who are looking at the positive effects of living in the now. You will appear to be more vibrant, more "in the know" and like someone who is already achieving their dreams, instead of someone who is stumbling along on the path to their dreams.

Chapter 11:
Set up small and practical goals

Life is a perfect continuation of new and different phases. Just one thing which makes it perfectly enjoyable is its characteristics of being monotonous make it worth considering. It is because of this variability and monotony that one has to keep on planning and thinking about his upcoming goals and dreams. It is not necessary that the same goal prevails for the whole life of an individual, neither is it possible that all goals may get achieved. So it requires a strategic and thoughtful approach to plan out one's goals and dream. Planning strategically is even more challenging, that is why many of us lag behind our goals. The reason is our insane approach towards the planning of our goals and dreams

Never out reach your limits

On the venture of planning and crating your dreams and mission you may become overly passionate and enthusiastic. It is because on the planning table, one may not see the hurdles and the hardships, which will be on the way towards the goal. It is because of this reason that one may start thinking too large or out of the prospective, crafting larger goals. While planning or running behind your goals, keep one thing in mind that, being a human you have certain potentials and limits. You cannot cross those limits. If you try to go beyond your limits, the ultimate result will uncontrollable frustration and fatigue. As a result you may become incapable of even those goals which are achievable and practical. Another critical point may be the particular phase of lie, through which you are passing. A goal which looks unachievable at a particular point foo one's life may become, attainable after a small tome, depending upon the particular conditions and circumstances.

So describing your personal mission is even more critical than extending the efforts for achieving it. Efforts if directed in an accurate direction and streamlined way can lead you to attain your dreams more effectively and efficiently, otherwise you will keep on lingering from one place to another and the real purpose will remain unattained.

Comparison is not worthy

One of the biggest mistakes we undergo while on the course of our life is to compare ourselves with the others around, although we all are completely different entities, in term of competencies and life realities. In this comparison we leave behind the reality of difference between us and start focusing on the goals of others. While defining our goals we must be truly individualistic. What others have achieved in their lives, may not be useful or worthy for us. Not only the life circumstances differ, but the life needs also vary. What is proving to be beneficial in other's lie may come out to be a total disaster in your life, so you need to be extra cautious in setting up your goals. Make your own decisions, depending upon your customized needs, without comparing them with others.

See too small but permanent changes

The life goals and dreams may also refer to the incorporation of certain changes in your personal or professional lie. Many people fail in getting their dreams achieved, because their canvas for life achievements is too broad. So in the fulfillment of these broad areas of life requirements, they become over pressurized. One if the finest strategy is to make an effective strategy. Effective strategy does not entail that very large leaps must be undertaken. Go for small and permanent changes. Permanency of an achievement is the biggest sign of victory.

So work for permanent way outs. If your goal is making permanent impressions in your life, it will give you a lifelong advantage in the shape of motivation and passion.

Achievable goals increase the chances of triumph

We have been largely talking about the listing and crafting of missions, goals and dreams, which on wants to achieve in his life. We have been talking about this limiting only because, once you will pick accurately you will get the right outcomes. When you are on your way towards the choice of your goals, you must be realistic. Having a proper knowledge about the life realities and your potentials, you will be better able to get success. One of the greatest benefits of having the practical goals is the motivation attached to the achievement. When one gets an initial success, it can serve as a greatest motivator to achieve larger and harder goals. In the initial phase if one gets, too unrealistic, the initial thing which will be encountered is the failure. The initial failure may become a permanent source of fatigue and agony, resulting in a great chaos.

So while you are making up your mind to get ready for a challenge of life, you have to conduct a thorough analysis for all the forces and factors which will give a combined effect in making your triumph nearer.

Chapter 12:
Maintain a long run Strategy

"A dream is your creative vision for your life in the future. You must break out of your current comfort zone and become comfortable with the unfamiliar and the unknown"

The human life is no less than a miracle. Even from the pre historical periods, the life of humans has been full of challenges and struggles, in order to survive and continue the greatest blessings of nature, which is life. If man has been ignorant about his environmental facts and factors, he has never been on your way toward life you may have encountered a number of factors.

Perform a thorough analysis for your abilities

When you are on your way towards the achievement of your dreams and goals, a number of major potentials may help you to get your final destinations. But the major and the most crucial advantage live in your inner self. One of the major reasons people usually fail in achieving their desired goals and dreams, is their inability to follow a systematic approach. Systematic approach demands that e very step in one's life must be defined in a way which is helpful for the achievement of one's goal. Whether the goals are personal or professional, you need to upgrade your approach.

The foremost thing is to perform a thorough analysis of your personality and list down all the basic abilities and weaknesses you possess. It will enable you to get a realistic view of your position so that you can judge that what is needed to get to your dreams. Listing down the capacities and weaknesses is not the only y thing. You need to judge the level of each capacity. It will provide you a list of all those abilities in the form of ranking, so that you will be able to make out that which ability will help you more and which needs to polished and refined.

Be a motivator for yourself

All these abilities and competencies when listed and appreciated can serve as a big motivator for an individual. On your way towards goal and missions, you need to be enthusiastic and passionate. It is not possible for even the most enthusiastic person that he remains with the same level of energy and passion, throughout his journey of goals. On your route of missions, you may possess multiple goals and missions. Some of these goals may be short term and some may be long term. So if you are catering multiple goals, you need to be continuously motivated to keep your journey continuous and long lasting.

Motivate yourself by appreciating your abilities. Whenever you feel low on the continuum of passion, start utilizing your abilities and talents

Be optimistic

Possessing the abilities is not a simple fact. Everyone possesses some or many abilities which may be useful in the achievement of the goals in one way or the other. The course of achieving your goals is not a simple one. If you have the long term goals, you need to be determined for a longer duration and you have to keep yourself passionate. Even if you find a hardship or failure in the course, the only thing which can keep you going is the power of optimism. It is such a divine and powerful tool that even the hardest of the journey can be easily passed using this extraordinary tool of achievement.

Optimism does not mean that one becomes over confident or unrealistic about the outcomes of a situation. It demands that one should not be over cautious or gloomy about a situation. The hardship or failure faced must be looked upon as a test of one's ability to withstand the challenges of life, not as the force for letting the individual down.

Stick to your abilities

On your way towards the hardships of life and achievement of different goals, if you are not actively aware of your abilities, your journey may become far more hard and tough. But if you have a full knowledge about the major abilities in your personality, you can use them for a number of different varying circumstances. Not having knowledge about your capabilities you may get to lose them with the passage of time. So in your struggle towards the goals and achievements you may lose abilities because you may have overlooked them, try to refine your abilities is such a way that all your abilities become a permanent part of your personality so that you never get short of these abilities because of ignorance. So if nature has bestowed you with some abilities try to make use of them at the utmost level so that you may become strong and successful with the passage of time. You will then need no any other help or support from anyone else.

Utilize your abilities to the fullest potential

Knowing about the abilities is just not enough. Penning the abilities and utilizing them to the fullest demand that we focus on each and every stance where a particular ability may be utilized. When you will be using your competencies over and over again, there are many chances that the competency gets polished into a fine talent. If you do not use your talent to the maximum level, you are actually making your destination even farther from your life. These are your abilities which can make your journey easy and simple. So you are suggested to make optimum use of your talents and strengths.

Never overlook your key potentials

There are many different ways in which your one can overlook his or her potentials. One reason may be the extreme fatigue, which is extracted from the pressure of achieving the life's goals and dreams. One becomes so involved in running after the results, that he or she becomes ignorant about the useful means of achieving these goals. Another reason may be the negative perspective of our personality. We start focusing on our weaknesses, and put an implicit mask on the availability of our potentials. So if you want to be a successful person in life you need to get fully involved in fighting or your dreams.

Chapter 13:
Prioritize your life goals

Prioritize your life goals, and find yourself to reach at maximum potential of your life

One's pulley of life weighs on two distinctive poles. One is to maximize the things and other is to minimize the things. This play of minimization-maximization actually lets the life to remain at a neutral stunt. Now, it depends on person that how he/she ponders his priorities. A successful person is the one who knows how to prioritize his/her goals.

Prioritization can't be fanatical. You would have to be practical and realistic in your goal. Just doing imaginations that what you can do and what you cannot do can never let you to reach the hill of prioritization. You must have to be clear in your vision and mission. Remove all ambiguities and be sensible. Clear your ways of success by prioritizing your life goals.

A quick guide to prioritize your life goals:

Life is progressive. It never remains static on a single pillar. The more supportive your life pillars are the more you will lead to the ladder of success. The settled goals are actually the pillars of success. They can change your failures and can convert your "failures" in to success. Let's clear the confusion and get a clear vision in setting your life term goals:

Arrange your life goals on Licker's scale:

Licker is the popped test constructer who introduces the measuring tool of goals. His scale contains the units from 1 to 7, or from 1-11. For sake of prioritizing your goals for long term

50

success, you may start arranging your goals on this scale. Let say, you are having 10 goals is your life. Tick 1 as "the goal most significant in your life", 2 as second most important goals of life, and so on.

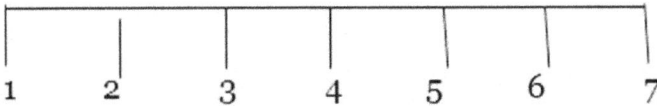

The game of preferences:

The prioritization of life goals is the game of preferences. YOU will label your goal in accord of your fondness. The goals those are more appealing for you would be kept at the top of your scale while those which are least appealing would be kept at the bottom.

Assemble your goals on time forecast:

Another good way of prioritizing your life goals is to assemble the on the basis of time forecast. A man can be multi tasked. But don't try to poke your nose in so many tasks simultaneously that are difficult to tackle. Be sharp and give a good hierarchy to your life term goals. The excellent solution is to pose goals, look at their preferences demand and accomplish them within frame of time forecaster like:

- 1 week

- 1 months

- 1 year

- 5 years

Look at your settled goal and fit them in the frame of time. Now challenge yourself to accomplish such tasks either by hook or by Crooke within fixed frame of time.

Find answer of questions to prioritize your life goals:

Answering to the mandatory questions is really important for sake of prioritizing your goal. Such answering will help you to confront what is most important up to what is least important for you. Be quick in your perceptions. The significant questions that you have to answer embraces:

- ✓ What are the basic goals of my life?

- ✓ How I can arrange my life goals from range of most important to least important?

- ✓ Which life goals are of long term usage for me?

- ✓ Which life goals are temporary beneficial?

- ✓ Which life goals when prioritize can peak up your head with proud and success?

- ✓ Which life goals are linear to the values of my society?

- ✓ Is there any set of goals which are mountable under my own hand?

- ✓ Am I arranging goal on social "should" or it is based on my internal will?

- ✓ Am I capable to stir these goals on my own behalf?

- ✓ Would I like to work on these goals?

- ✓ Are these life stunning goals are motivating for me or not?

- ✓ How I confirm goals on basis of their importance?

- ✓ How I will jump up to the ladder of success through the confirmed goals?

Let's make final hierarchy:

The final hierarchy aims to pet your goals. You have to give a final shape to your goals. You may follow the below plan chart and start putting your life goals in terms of your prioritization:

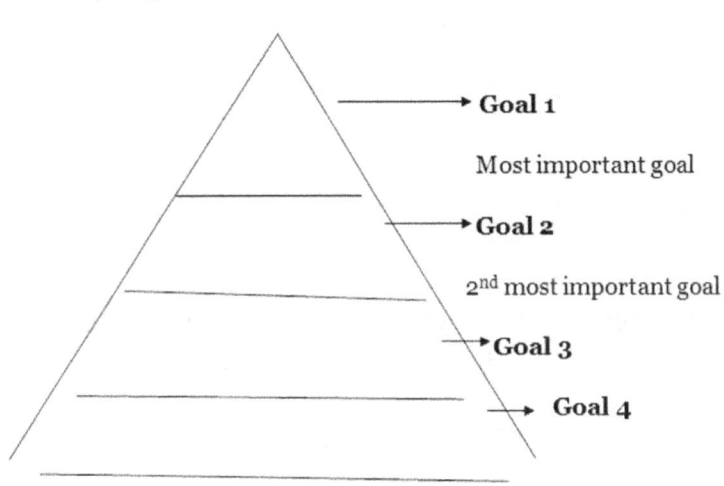

Shape your life by prioritizing your goals:

In the present digital globe adoption of old rules is really a foolish task. Now you would have to grasp your routine by the machine of your own hand. If you want to reach the sky of success then you would have to be sharp enough to tackle your life term goals.

Draw "enter/exit" by your own pen of mission:

Start tackling your life in terms of your prioritized goal. Give edges to the time of your life. Draw opening doors as the doors of success. Close all those doors that are hauling and are creating hurdles to success

For sake of accomplishing your task with perfection, you may give a stage wise pecking order to your goals as:

Stage one - the list & the beginning draw

Stage two – highlight most important goals

Stage three – give schedule to the life goals

Stage four – start underlining the "gained goals" and the "Remaining goals".

Golden secretive rules for prioritizing your life goals:

Here are some golden rules that can help you to prioritize your goals perfectly. With these enigmatic rules you can set your goals, can prioritize them and can get success in your hands:

Rule # 1: Fix the goals which are motivating for you

Rule # 2: Select smart goals which are specific, measurable, & attainable

Rule # 3: Make an action plan for your prioritized goals

Rule # 4: Start working on your settled goals

Rules # 5: Get success.

Critical evaluation:

You can make your prioritized goal as the "key to success". Avoid the goals which are ambiguous, very much time taking and out of reach. Never leave the edge of patience while working on your prioritized goals.

Chapter 14:
Get a habit of appreciating your achievements

Habits are actually the stunning parts of one's personality. They reflect the actual nature of person. Good habit/Bad habit works like the head in leading success of a person. So, wisdom is to become the mother of your habits. Give birth to good habits, grow them well and make your life popping in the world of victory.

Get the habit of appreciating your achievement:

Have you ever noticed how a little kid learns to behave accurately in one's situation? How he comes to know what to do and what not to do in a particular scenario? According to B.F Skinner, reinforcement molds and modifies one's behavior. It is appreciation which increases the likelihood of a child to re-do the demanding behavior. Means "appreciation" is a proven of strengthen one's desirable behavior. So, if you want to strengthen your habit of achievement in your life then do take the help of "appreciation".

Reinforce your abilities:

Reinforcement is the dramatic aspect of appreciation. Start reinforcing your abilities. Back-up yourself on your gaining's. Set a rewarding system for you. You will feel it will amuse yourself. You will start finding a joy an inner satisfaction in doing what you can.

Dramatize your achievements:

"Imaginations" are the roots which actually gives growth to success. So, start dramatizing your achievements. It will show you a path towards success. So, start dramatizing your achievements. And you will see these achievements will starts happening in the real life.

Dig out achievement's routs by yourself:

A man is a constructor of his abilities. God gave mind to man and thus leave him responsible of using it. So, be the one to open routes of achievements for you. Dig the routes of success for you.

Back-up your ability to control the ticks of clock:

Believe on it that everybody has same 24 hours of the day. It is up to a man that how he makes it worthy for him. So, believe on it that ticks of clock are under your control. You can make them precious. You can make end of your day a golden end for you.

Acknowledge your achievements:

Don't be like those boozy people who just maximize their failures. Such foolish people keep poking their nose on what they have not in their hands. They keep bothering about what is far away from them, what is non-attainable for them and what is behind their reach. They just break their heads on those sparkling things which they can just see in their dreams.

Being a one among them is not a wise decision. Just take a faith on quote "All glitters are not that gold". Be appreciative and indebt what you have. Start acknowledging all, what you have gained in your life. Make your eye ball expanded on what you have gained and what you are going to gain. Keep foresight but don't put this prudence on top.

Be appreciative:

Back up your gains! Start weighing your own self in front of others and thus show other the door of your abilities and skills. Start owing your own name. Be the one to confront others what you are? What makes you different from others? What is highly fascinating and appreciating in you? The world does not have enough time to go and to scratch what you are. It will only believe in what you will show on the screen. So, be wise and shows the gorgeous side of you.

Realize that you are important:

Start finding the reality of yourself. Look at your hands and find can't they write? Can't they take the things in them? Look at your feet! Can't you go far distance with them? Start analyzing yourself and abilities. What your mind is and how you can take work from it. Automatically you will be able to recognize your importance. You will look you have many of thrilling and chilling abilities. You just have to buff up them all.

Appreciate what you have done:

Most people keep saying that they did nothing in their lives. Okay if you are one among them then I challenge you that you are wrong. If you say you did nothing in your life then I am going to ask you little questions:

- Have you never washed your face?

- Have you never displaced from your place?

- Do you not even know how to write A up to Z?

- Are you sure you never move your hand?

I am damn sure your answer will be "BIG NO". Then if you can move your hand, you can move from one place to another then you can do many things in your life. So, start appreciating what you have done and start striving what you have not done.

If you say yes you have washed you face many times, and of course you can move from one place to another. And for sure, you can write from A to Z and you can give any sort of movement to your hand then look! You are capable of doing if not all but partial works of this world. If you are educated you can be receptionist, you can be writer, advertiser, lawyer and more. If you are uneducated still you can do many tasks like driving, tailoring, vowing and so on. So, start putting light on what you can do.

You are golden and you can make everything gold!

Start believing on yourself. Nobody can be as much sincere with you as you can be with yourself. Don't underestimate your powers. Start working on your skills and abilities. Just focus on your good works. Consider you are golden and you are a shining star. You can shine and can give light to others as well.

Look in the mirror and confidently concede your achievements:

Start taking responsibilities! Go and stand in front of the mirror. Start analyzing what you have achieved and what is still in progress to achieve. Start giving feedback to yourself. Just make it amazing that you are an enlighten candle.

Chapter 15:
Never overdo your efforts

"Efforts will release its reward only when you refuse to quit"

Life is a beautiful collection of different shades. The different colors and sides of the picture present a new challenge, after every new day. So we humans need to get well equipped with all its realities and facts so that we can understand such a broader picture of life. We can never get rid of the struggle and efforts needed to get through this challenging life, yet the only thing we can do is to get a proactive orientation towards all the life realities. In this life the multiple life arenas can make you go into an ever going exercise of life struggle and in this struggle we may sometime loose our own identity and inner peace. All you need is a wise approach towards your dreams.

When we talk about the discourse of one's life dreams, we may get a number of different facts. Not all goals are related to on aspect of life. As life changes the priorities change. In the childhood we may be least bothered about the harsh realities of life, including the financial and economic pressures, but as the pages of life are turned, many new and challenging realities may get highlighted.

Save your stamina for harder ventures

Many people are not the true strategic thinkers. They do not plan the life challenges according to their list of priorities or importance. When they encounter even a minor issue, they become defensive and put on the hardest approach to deal with it. This is not a wise approach. When you start exerting your highest efforts on the least important tasks, you are actually wasting your valuable resources, which nature has blessed you in the shape of talents and competencies. So you never know that when in life you encounter a challenge which is more demanding than these unimportant tasks. So you have to prepare for the more strenuous tasks, for that you need to save your crucial stamina and energy. In this way you can exert your efforts for more challenging tasks, and dealing with less important issues will be helpful.

You may encounter even harder ventures

Life is totally a surprise. One fine morning you may get something which was totally out of your thinking, or on the other hand you may get such a challenge which was never thought by you. In both cases, your ability to face the unexpected and unknown challenge may let you get through it firmly. It is a reality that no one in this life can remain aloof from the hardships of life, so whatever he may encounter he has to put efforts. Our point here is to make you ready for the life ventures in a way that all your dreams can come true and you may not feel any sense of fatigue. Although life is a notion of continuous effort and exertion, but once we put our efforts in an organized way, we are able to maintain a perfect balance. In the initial years of your personal and professional life the type of challenges may be different than the ones you encounter in the later parts of your life. People usually get interconnected goals when they become involved in the family matters, so it is essential duty of everyone to get him ready for the harder tasks. If you make use of your stamina for irrelevant facts, you are actually putting a hindrance to your potentials. Life can pose an even greater challenge at any time, so make sure that you are ready for it.

Do not put all your eggs in one basket

While preparing for your goals and dreams, make one thing certain that you have a proper plan and layout for the systematic oath of your life. Most of us have the multiple boundaries of our lives, from daily household life to the routine work life. But all these arenas of life are equally important. When you are planning about all these domains of life, you have to follow a very multidimensional approach. If one set his goals pertaining to a particular arena of life are at stake, make sure that the other one is perfectly saved. In this way you can easily avoid the complete chaos in life. If you do not follow this approach, you will get a completely muddled and gloomy. Try to be a multitasking person, yet the wise approach is to save your one ground of opportunities. Keeping all your dreams and goals at stake is not a wise approach.

Think about the survival of your soul

When you are extending all your energy and efforts to make your dreams come true, all you need is the attainment of your goals and dreams. But in this course of hardships and struggles, you may sometimes, forget your own self and it can put a permanent impressions of hardships on your soul. To strive and struggle for one's goals is no matter a brave and a wise approach, yet going in to this struggle, too far is never a positive and wise approach. All you need is to get a course of action which can maintain your inner self as well as help you attain your goals and reams. The efforts which are highly over exerting can make you lose the real purpose of life, and you may get into an ever going cycle of struggle and effort. Extending efforts for your dreams is surely needed, yet you have to keep a balance. Stop this vicious cycle when it goes beyond a certain limit.

Chapter 16:
Time is money, so schedule yourself

Time is money – So cash it and hunt success in your feet

What you think about time? Is it having enough plenty to waste it, to squander it and to make misuse of it? If you uncover the pages of unsuccessful people, then you will find "exploitation of time" the most. They mistake in understanding the worth of time.

Every person in this world is facing the same transitions in time. The same morn welcomes every man, the same afternoon shake hand with everybody and the same night comes for each and every person of this world. Then bother your mind where the difference comes? Why some people are at the top of success while others are still striving? The one and only reason that will dominate the answer will be "the usage of time".

Great people tackle the time greatly. They think and take every moment of life as the most worthy moment. Such people believe in reasoning. They work on an abstract level and cater to answer how to utilize the time? What activity can make their time beneficial for them? They kick out those activities which are bogus and free of output.

Draw a memo of your life:

If you want to be successful, and then believe it "your life is a Performa". You will hold agendas over it and will fill this Performa with the actions of your life. Develop memo for your life. This memo must be systematic and organized. Think how you can settle down the tasks equally. Your memo can be your guide! The best guide that can direct you how to take start, how to take move and how to reach an end of success.

Put ticks of clock under your control:

If you know the reality that every man has the same 24 hours a day. Now it is his own choice how he utilizes it. Such 24 hours can be passed like the routine of the day, with doing nothings. And such 24 hours can be passed by blissful activities. So, be a good decision maker and decide how you are going to utilize such 24 hours of the day. Be pathetic & miser is its usage. Utilize every bit of your time is fruitful activities.

Be purposive:

Shun off extra activities from your schedule. Kick them off like the hurdles of life. Be wise and start focusing on what is good for you. Avoid mechanistic approach and focus on purposive approach. As Carl Jung said "a man is purposive, what he did has passed away, he has many opportunities to avail in coming days". He is the one who opposes the "mechanistic concept" of Freud. Sigmund Freud was of the view" a person is mechanistic and he remains adhered to what he did in past".

So, don't be foolish and be purposive. Avoid what you have done worthlessly. Make your future bright. If you will keep grasping what wrong you did, then you can never come out of your past and you can never cash your new coming golden time.

Create your time:

Be a good creator to be a good successor. Learn how to create the good time for you. If time is not companioning you, enable yourself to make time your companion. Learn how to convert bad time into good time. Start chasing the moments of your time like:

5 am to 7 am ------ Activity – 1

8 am – 10 am ----- Activity – 2

11 am – 12 am ---- Activity - 3

And so on. This is how you can manage your time and can utilize it worthy.

Don't move blindly:

If you will remain unscheduled, and will not schedule your time then for sure you will move like a blind person. Just take an example, if you are non-scheduled and you don't know what to do and when to do then your schedule will be like:

	Time	Time	Time	Time
	7 – 8 am	9 – 10 am	11 – 12 am	1- 2 pm
Day 1:	Activity A	Activity B	Activity D	Activity C
Day 2:	Activity C	Activity E	Activity A	Activity B
Day 3:	Activity B	Activity C	Activity D	Activity A
Day 4:	Activity E	Activity D	Activity A	Activity C

Just notice and give a review, do you understand what is managed in the above the schedule? When you even can't understand what is written in one paragraphed schedule, then how you can work on it? It will let all your efforts to go in vein. You may focus that in above schedule; a person with no theme has also inserted activity E uncertain in some of the days. So, what you will call it? A good schedule or an excellent foolishness!

Start multiplying your profit with hours of the day:

Manage your time to multiply your profits. Establish your settings in a way that you can worth all those activities that give cash to you. Make your mental frame in a way that you can do something unique and perfect.

Be the slave of time:

When you will make yourself a slave of time, then you will see grasping the mastery of the world. Welcome this master slave relation and you will see that how rapidly success will touch your feet.

Hunt your time logistically:

Don't pass the time just for killing it! Fit it logistically into the blocks of works. Create an importance for the time and you will feel a craving of success in your heart. Start finding logics. When you will start moving on an abstract level, then you will find your fanatical dream starts becoming true.

Time is money! So start cashing it. It is an astounding key to success. You can hunt success with ease if you know how to make the time worthy. Either become the slave of time or become the slave of this world. So, come to know how you can manage and utilize your time with best effort and with excellent output.

Chapter 17:
Dig out some lessons from your failures

"The season of failure is the best time for sowing the seeds of success"

Throughout this book we have been talking about the life dreams and goals. We have provided a detailed guideline for our readers that how can they make best use of their potentials to get the benefit of the power of now and make their life successful in all arenas of life. All you need is a positive approach towards all phases of life. When we talk about the life and the dreams we pursue in this life, we talk about opportunities, we ponder upon our strengths and we investigate the enthusiasm. But only a few of us start following a proactive approach by giving a due attention towards our failures. For us the most disliked portion of our discourse is the rise of some failure. So either we don't talk about failure or push them into the backyard of our life.

However, failure can polish your struggle for the attainment of your dreams and goals.

Failures are lifelong lessons

Imagine a runner who is practicing for a Marathon and encounters a fall in his practice session. After these initial falls, his instructor teaches him to avoid falling by losing the balance. So the failures in his practice session make him learn a lot for his contest of Marathon. You can use the similar stance in the course of your life, when every coming day poses a new challenge. Going through these challenges you may come to know a number of your weaknesses and the resulting failures. But if you want to pursue your dreams, you cannot make these failures, a hurdle for your dreams. All you can do is to follow a systematic approach and make a record of all the failures encountered in your life and make use of them, as useful lessons for the rest of your life. All you can do is to dig out the benefit from your failures. Failures can be your real time instructors, which have the greatest potential to teach.

Modifying your talents, need a hard core lesson

We have been focusing on the use of abilities sand capacities, in the best possible way. But all capacities are not full to your potential from the very beginning. They need to be polished and modified with the passage of time, so that they can be used in a variety of circumstances. Using your talents and potentials in the life is like a hit and trial exercise, but once you have a full knowledge about your potentials you can use them in varying situations. One such way of polishing your skills is to learn from your failures. All you need is to take every failure and make it a case of learning by understanding that what particular characteristics and abilities were needed to avoid this particular failure. In this way you will be able to make use of your failure as a mode of modifying your talents. Convert your failure into a learning opportunity and maintain a steady balance between lifelong pending decisions and those dreams which need to be achieved within a short duration of time. The opportunities can turn fruitful only and only if one has the potential to get the maximum benefit out of them, otherwise the whole thing gets ruined, within no time. All you need is a perfect match of strategic approach and the wider perspective of your life so that you may not be left with any hard feelings about your dreams and the related potentials. You can get the maximum out of it.

What you are thinking as a failure may be a success in the long run

The greatest mistake we execute in achieving a goal is to give up our struggle. Sometimes an individual covers a hard and tough passage very smoothly and one small failure misguides him from his real purpose and him stop following his dreams. This is the most unproductive approach. If a small failure makes you alert about the forthcoming big hurdle, you can utilize the failure as a big ladder towards the success. We sometimes think that if we are getting the hardships in the short run, we should quit following our dreams. However, the hardships encountered today can be a source of pleasure and joy in the long run. So whenever you are devising a plan for achieving your dreams, make yourself oriented towards the long run so that you can think in a wider spectrum and you can easily make the choice which will be beneficial in achieving your dreams.

That's not the end of the story

Many people quit after the first mistake and this is where they commit the first mistake. Failures are good as long as you keep going. Quitting because of the failures is a cowards approach. Every beginning needs a solid drive and for that purpose the lessons learnt from the failures, can serve as your guide for a new venture and new journey towards your dreams and passions.

One needs to bring a permanent plan out for making your dreams come true , for that purpose a real systematic approach will surely workout otherwise it will make your all plans and dreams get gloomy in the struggles of life.

Conclusion

As you reflect on the power of now, there are certain things that should come to light. The first is a belief in your own consciousness, and how you view yourself and your abilities. Setting your mind to achieving your dreams by taking action in the now involves a process, and some organization.

It is important that you state what your goals are and become clear about them. Following which, you need to set aside the necessary time to fully focus on your plans, and how you can bring them to fruition. You do this, by creating a detailed plan, which will outline the steps that you need to take, how you will control all your emotions and how you can measure your end results.

A large part of being able to take action and appreciate the power of now involves taking full control of your emotions, and not allowing your mind to run away with you. You should be able to easily eliminate doubt, fear and worry, so that you set yourself free to have your dreams come true.

As much as you can use the help of others, and draw inspiration from them, you cannot transfer the responsibility in your life onto the shoulders of other people. You should be accountable for yourself, how you treat others, how you react to situations and what you speak into your own mind so that you can achieve your dreams.

Changing your mind set is important to taking action now. Rather than seeing the glass half empty, you have the opportunity to see it as half full. Take that chance NOW, and move closer to your dreams faster than you thoughts was possible.

www.ingramcontent.com/pod-product-compliance
Lightning Source LLC
Chambersburg PA
CBHW070607290526
45790CB00002B/823